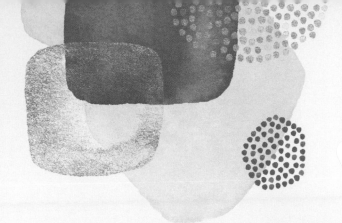

RESILIENCY GUIDES

GROW YOUR GRATITUDE

A Guided Journal for Creating a Joyful Life

Janine Wilburn

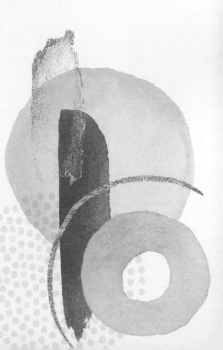

WEST
MARGIN
PRESS

The Gift of Gratitude

To be grateful is to give oneself an extraordinary gift

A gift that shines light where there is darkness

Brings happiness where there is sadness

Healing where there is hurt

Hope where there is despair

To be grateful is joyful

To be grateful is giving

To be grateful is compassionate, wise and forgiving

To be grateful is everlasting.

—J. Wilburn

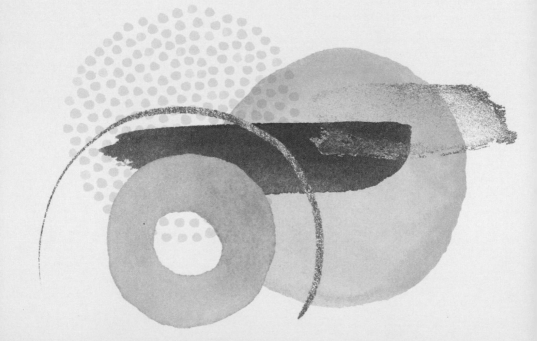

This journal belongs to

_____

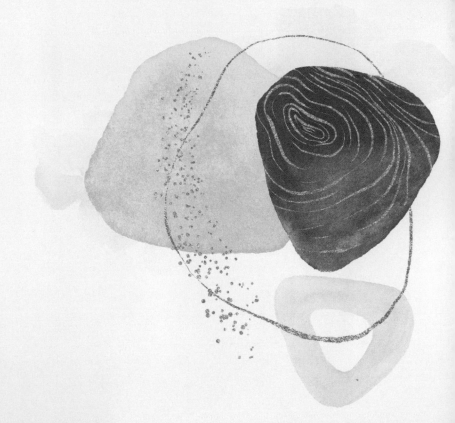

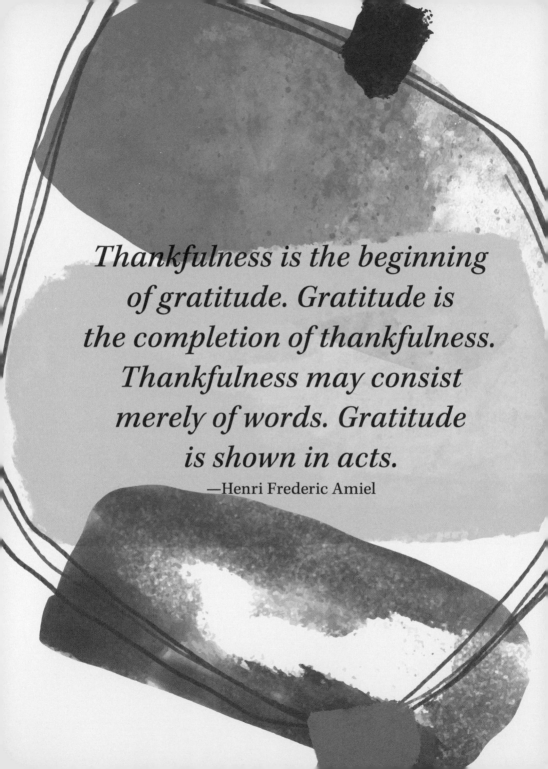

Thankfulness is the beginning of gratitude. Gratitude is the completion of thankfulness. Thankfulness may consist merely of words. Gratitude is shown in acts.

—Henri Frederic Amiel

CONTENTS

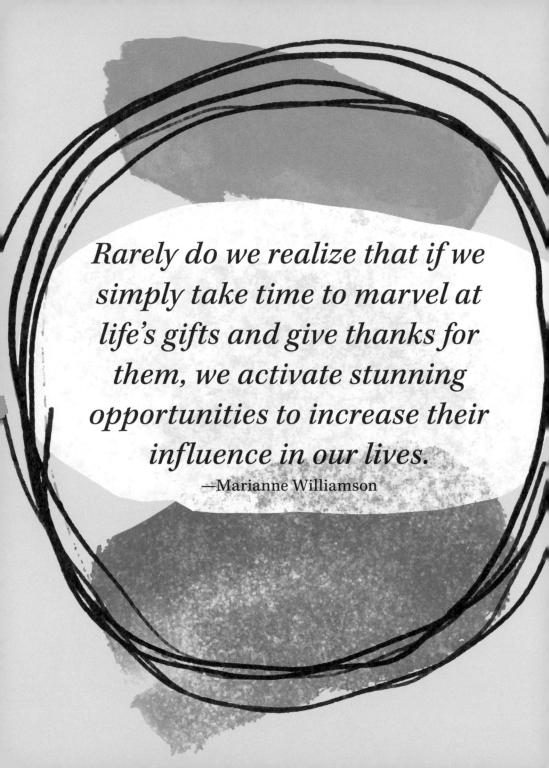

Rarely do we realize that if we simply take time to marvel at life's gifts and give thanks for them, we activate stunning opportunities to increase their influence in our lives.

—Marianne Williamson

INTRODUCTION

The Greatness of Gratitude

Gratitude helps you create the life you want.

As popular as gratitude is, it is often misunderstood. Many believe it is just a feeling that comes when someone is kind to you or something nice happens to you. Or some equate it to finding the silver linings in life. These are aspects and qualities of gratitude, but they do not speak to the entirety of gratitude.

Gratitude is actually a state of being. Gratitude is a state of grace that provides comfort, direction, and perspective even in the face of great challenges. It is a powerful tool that allows one to stand in the face of disappointment, ill health, loss, and even death with strength and resiliency.

According to Dr. Robert Emmons at the University of California at Davis, gratitude is a choice: "It means that we sharpen our ability to recognize and acknowledge the giftedness of life. It means that we make a conscious decision to see blessings instead of curses. It means that our internal reactions are not determined by external forces. That gratitude is a conscious decision does not imply that it is an easy decision... while gratitude is pleasant, it is not easy."

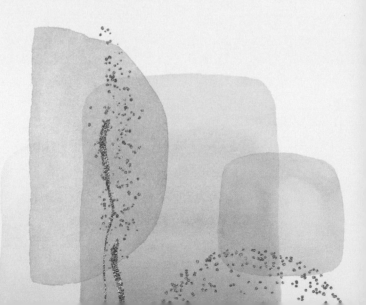

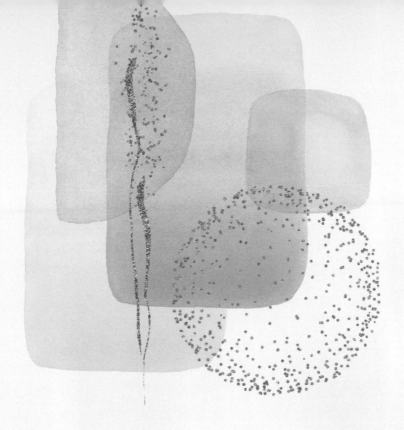

Rather, gratitude is a highly efficient tool that supports our mental, emotional, physical, and spiritual bodies. The power of gratitude is almost incomprehensible as it seems to be such a simple act of acknowledgment. However, when facing overwhelming difficulties and deep loss, reaching for gratitude can feel more challenging than climbing Mount Everest.

That is why it is critical to understand that gratitude is not just an emotion—it is a tool that brings peace, even happiness, to pain and loss. Gratitude can help us melt away challenges by positively shifting our perspective and our sense of well-being. In fact, studies show gratitude can be used to help with mood swings, anxiety, post-traumatic stress, and even sleep challenges.

Why I Created This Journal

Resiliency plays a critical role in my daily life and in my family's life. Twenty-four years ago, I was in a serious car accident. I experienced severe spinal injuries, including spinal cord compression in my neck and additional disc damage throughout my spine. The prognosis: it was only a matter of time before I would lose movement from the neck down. It was at this juncture in my life when I first encountered a distinction in neuroscience called neuroplasticity, through Sharon Begley's book *Train Your Mind, Change Your Brain* and her exploration of Dr. Richard Davidson's research at the University of Wisconsin–Madison (my alma mater). I read and reread the book, and then studied everything I could find on the subject. I knew there were answers in the science to help me heal when most of my doctors and health care practitioners no longer believed it was possible.

I began to engage and develop daily practices that eventually were identified through research as the building blocks of resiliency. The results were overwhelmingly positive. My pain started to diminish, and sleep was available for a few hours at a time. I discovered that by being creative I could significantly minimize my pain, so I became a visual artist, even though I had limited use of my hands and arms at the time.

I dug deeper into observing, monitoring, and utilizing my thoughts to enhance my healing, and combined that knowledge and intention to create my many daily practices. In pursuit of a "cure," I found so much more. I learned the importance of love when dealing with hardship. I learned love comes in so many shapes and sizes: forgiveness, gratitude, kindness, creativity, acts of service, authentic listening, compassion, daily practices, prayer, meditation, yoga, still and quiet moments, exercise, and healthy eating.

My favorite go-to tool is gratitude, as I can use it anywhere at any time. It has gotten me through incredibly challenging times. If my gratitude journal is not nearby, I will say gratitude statements out loud or in my mind, helping me to deal with everything from physical pain and emotional upset to mental fatigue and overwhelm. Whether the difficulties are aspects of my personal life or our collective lives, gratitude helps relieve the stress.

Although my sought-after "return to normal" has not materialized, I am deeply grateful that I can walk and move without assistance. On this twenty-four-year journey, I have learned so much, gained so much knowledge and maybe a little wisdom. I learned a new definition of hope—our only opportunity for control. I learned that real, open-hearted connection is critical; that gratitude is one of our greatest tools; and that being of service is one of our greatest gifts. I learned to never stop trying and to never give up. I learned to appreciate every day and work to be present and conscious in the moment.

I have so much—my family who inspires me every day, my dedicated teachers who continue to support me, the people who allow me to be of service in their lives, my daily practices, and the many, many aspects of love. All this helps me to resiliently create and shape a life I love and am passionate about even during the most painful moments. I learned we never really know what the next moment or twenty-four years have in store for us; however, with our minds and our gratitude practices, we can make it something special.

How to Use This Book

Grow Your Gratitude is a guided journal for you to explore and experience the power of gratitude as it helps you build resiliency. Every page is filled with engaging prompts and creative activities which show you how to bring gratitude into your daily life.

Gratitude is most powerful when it becomes part of your routine. Creating a gratitude practice by journaling everyday gratitudes or writing daily gratitude lists helps build resiliency; and on those really hard days you can then read and reread your gratitudes from previous days. So pick a time of day to do your gratitude statements and try to stick to it. Some people find starting their days with their gratitude practice sets a strongly positive tone for the day. Others prefer to write their gratitude statements during the day. Many choose to write their gratitude statements in the evening before going to sleep. Research reveals many people self-report better sleep after doing their gratitudes before bed.

There are two ways to use this journal to bring gratitude into your daily life. One way is to start at the beginning of the journal and make your way from the first page to the last page. The other approach is to open the journal and fill out the two pages that you land on. The journal has been designed so that the pages on the left engage you with many different sources to create your gratitude statements, while the pages on the right allow you to capture your personal gratitude experience for that day. Regardless of which approach you choose, filling out both pages every day not only brings and records the benefits you experience that day, but will also help you develop a gratitude practice by the time you complete the journal.

Don't be surprised when at times you may not feel like you

want to write anything, or that you are even irritated by the thought. That is why there are examples in every section to make it easier in those moments. On those days commit to yourself to write at least five statements. You can be grateful for anything, and you don't have to experience feeling grateful when you write your gratitude statements. People regularly report that they end up doing many more than five statements, and feeling better mentally, emotionally, and even physically.

As the days pass, notice your gratitude practice move from something new to something routine. Eventually, the routine will become a habit, and it will be harder not to do your gratitude practice than to do it. Finally, the habit becomes a daily ritual, and that gratitude practice will last you a lifetime. It will be helpful when you're upset, angry, or hurt as well as when you are happy. When developing your gratitude practice, you can express gratitude over things that have happened, and create gratitude intentions for things you would like to have happen. There is not a right way or wrong way to be grateful or to do gratitude. The most valuable thing is to do it!

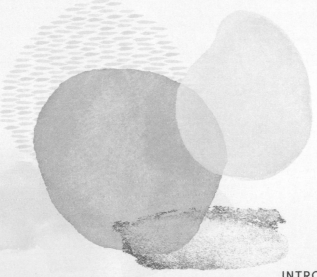

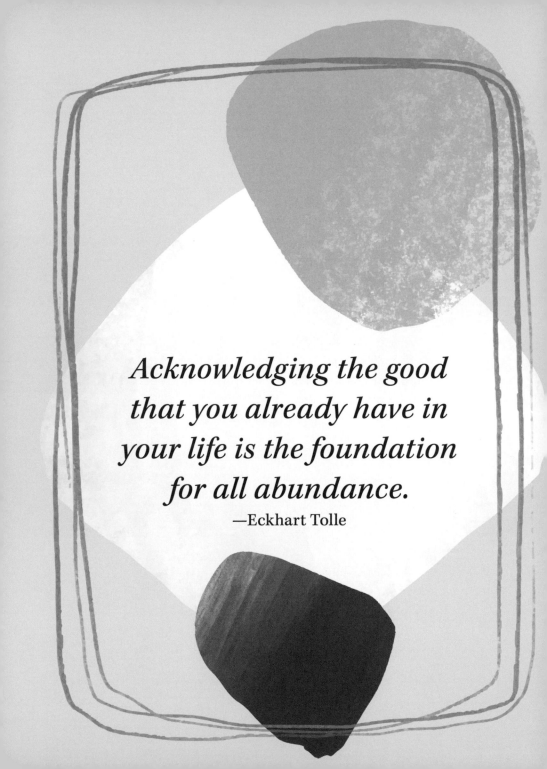

*Acknowledging the good
that you already have in
your life is the foundation
for all abundance.*

—Eckhart Tolle

FINDING GRATITUDE

Locating Your Gratitude

Look closely at aspects of your everyday life and find the people, places, and things you like, enjoy, and appreciate. Look and recognize all that contributes to your day in big ways and, equally important, in small ways. For example, when someone steps back to let you take the place in line in front of them or relinquishes a parking spot to you, or when a stranger smiles at you for no apparent reason. Take mental note and then express gratitude for them, their action, or both. As you fill out the pages in this journal, notice where your gratitude lives within you—how it feels and where you feel it.

PEOPLE I AM GRATEFUL FOR

Acknowledge your gratitude for the people who make a difference in your life. They can be family members, friends, colleagues, coworkers, neighbors, teachers and mentors, frontline workers, service providers, and even strangers. Write their names, and if you'd like, add what specifically you are grateful for beside each name. The statements can be as general or specific as you choose. For example: *I am grateful for my long-time friend Laurie always being there for me.*

Family who I am grateful for...

I am grateful for _____

I am grateful for _____

I am grateful for _____

I am grateful for _____

I am grateful for _____

Friends who I am grateful for...

I am grateful for _____

I am grateful for _____

I am grateful for _____

I am grateful for _____

I am grateful for _____

Colleagues & teammates who I am grateful for...

-
-
-
-
-

Coworkers who I am grateful for...

-
-
-
-
-

Mark where you feel your
gratitude today.

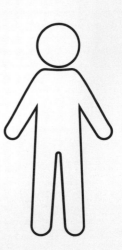

PEOPLE I AM GRATEFUL FOR

Think about and recognize people who have contributed to you in your life recently or in the past. Include their names and something specific they did for you. For example: *I am grateful for Professor Jim supporting my career ambitions through school and beyond.*

Teachers & mentors who I am grateful for...

I am grateful for _____

I am grateful for _____

I am grateful for _____

I am grateful for _____

I am grateful for _____

People in my community who I am grateful for...

I am grateful for _____

I am grateful for _____

I am grateful for _____

I am grateful for _____

I am grateful for _____

Frontline workers & health care professionals who I am grateful for...

-
-
-
-
-

Service providers who I am grateful for...

-
-
-
-

Mark where you feel your gratitude today.

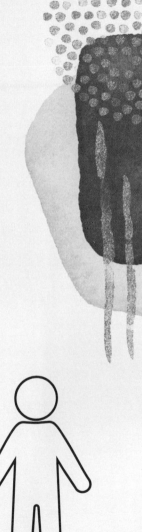

PLACES I AM GRATEFUL FOR

Acknowledge your gratitude for the places that give you comfort. For example, you can be grateful for your favorite chair you relax into. Or you can be grateful for the old oak tree that is outside where you live.

As I look around where I live, inside my space I am grateful for...

I am grateful for _____

I am grateful for _____

I am grateful for _____

I am grateful for _____

I am grateful for _____

As I look around where I live, outside my space I am grateful for...

I am grateful for _____

I am grateful for _____

I am grateful for _____

I am grateful for _____

I am grateful for _____

Restaurants, coffee shops, & stores I like to go to frequently...

-
-
-
-
-

Places where I go to relax and think...

-
-
-
-
-

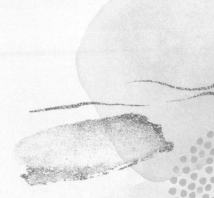

Mark where you feel your gratitude today.

BELONGINGS I AM GRATEFUL FOR

Identify belongings that are very special to you or hold important memories. It can be anything from your favorite socks or T-shirt to photos of loved ones.

Belongings that hold special memories...

I am grateful for _____

I am grateful for _____

I am grateful for _____

I am grateful for _____

I am grateful for _____

Belongings I am grateful to have every day...

I am grateful for _____

I am grateful for _____

I am grateful for _____

I am grateful for _____

I am grateful for _____

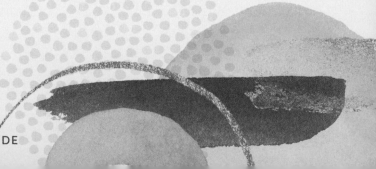

ACTIVITIES I AM GRATEFUL FOR

Take a moment to think about and recognize things you do in your regular life that you are grateful for being able to do. They could be activities you participate in outdoors and indoors.

Outside activities I enjoy...

-
-
-
-

Inside activities I enjoy...

-
-
-
-

Mark where you feel your gratitude today.

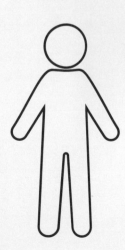

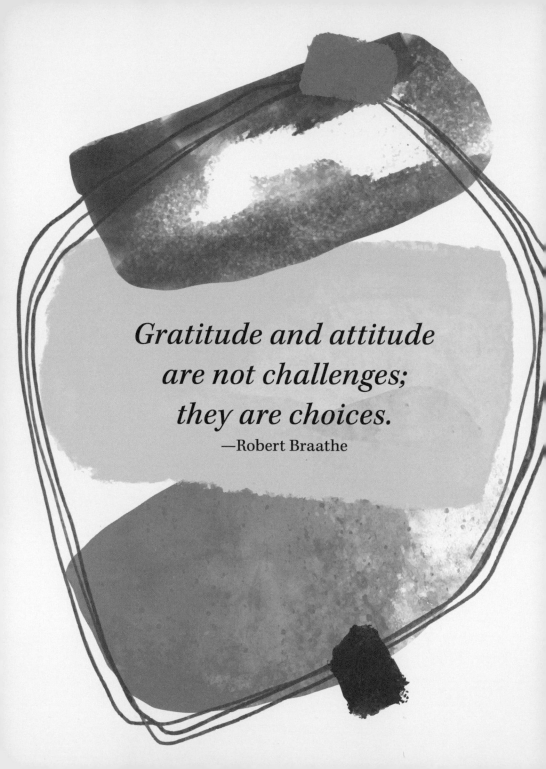

Gratitude and attitude are not challenges; they are choices.
—Robert Braathe

LIVING GRATITUDE

Immersing Yourself in Gratitude

Take a step back to remember and recognize the people, things, and events that have positively contributed to your life. Whether the contribution is big or small, recent or in the past, it is worth noting and acknowledging as it is helps teach us how to live in the greatness of gratitude.

PEOPLE IN MY LIFE I WILL ALWAYS BE GRATEFUL FOR

You can fill out this page in one sitting, or take your time adding to it whenever you wish. For example: *I am grateful for my art teacher who helped me find the artist in myself.*

I am grateful for _____

_____

I am grateful for _____

_____

I am grateful for _____

_____

I am grateful for _____

_____

I am grateful for _____

_____

I am grateful for _____

_____

I am grateful for _____

_____

TODAY'S GRATITUDE

Date _____

These are the people, things, and events that I am
grateful for today.

I am grateful for _____

_____

I am grateful for _____

_____

I am grateful for _____

_____

I am grateful for _____

_____

I am grateful for _____

_____

This is where I feel my gratitude today.

THINGS IN MY LIFE I WILL ALWAYS BE GRATEFUL FOR

You can fill out this page in one sitting, or take your time adding to it whenever you wish. For example: *I am grateful for learning my favorite sport, basketball.*

I am grateful for _____

_____

I am grateful for _____

_____

I am grateful for _____

_____

I am grateful for _____

_____

I am grateful for _____

_____

I am grateful for _____

_____

I am grateful for _____

_____

TODAY'S GRATITUDE

Date _____

These are the people, things, and events that I am grateful for today.

I am grateful for _____
_____

I am grateful for _____
_____

I am grateful for _____
_____

I am grateful for _____
_____

I am grateful for _____
_____

This is where I feel my gratitude today.

EVENTS IN MY LIFE THAT I WILL ALWAYS REMEMBER

You can fill out this page in one sitting, or take your time adding to it whenever you wish. For example: *I am grateful for visiting Venice during my trip to Italy.*

I am grateful for _____
_____

I am grateful for _____
_____

I am grateful for _____
_____

I am grateful for _____
_____

I am grateful for _____
_____

I am grateful for _____
_____

I am grateful for _____
_____

TODAY'S GRATITUDE

Date _____

These are the people, things, and events that I am grateful for today.

I am grateful for _____
_____

I am grateful for _____
_____

I am grateful for _____
_____

I am grateful for _____
_____

I am grateful for _____
_____

This is where I feel my gratitude today.

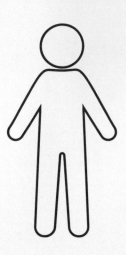

WHAT I AM GRATEFUL FOR OVER THE PAST YEAR

You can fill out this page in one sitting, or take your time adding to it whenever you wish. For example: *I am grateful for beginning to practice yoga last year.*

I am grateful for _____

_____

I am grateful for _____

_____

I am grateful for _____

_____

I am grateful for _____

_____

I am grateful for _____

_____

I am grateful for _____

_____

I am grateful for _____

_____

I am grateful for _____

_____

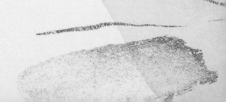

TODAY'S GRATITUDE

Date _____

These are the people, things, and events that I am grateful for today.

I am grateful for _____
_____

I am grateful for _____
_____

I am grateful for _____
_____

I am grateful for _____
_____

I am grateful for _____
_____

This is where I feel my gratitude today.

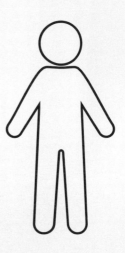

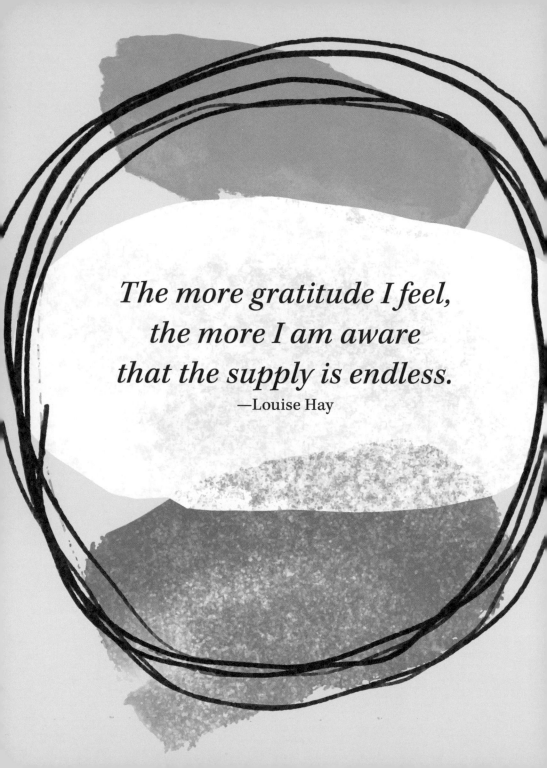

The more gratitude I feel,
the more I am aware
that the supply is endless.
—Louise Hay

CREATING GRATITUDE

Composing Gratitude Intentions

The gratitude statements you write in this section are different from the ones you just completed. Here, you will generate gratitude statements for what you desire in your life as if it currently exists. For example, if you are looking for a new place to live, you would write: *I am grateful for my new home.* Reread your gratitude intentions regularly to keep them in mind, and keep adding to them over time.

GRATITUDE INTENTIONS FOR MY DAILY LIFE

Close your eyes and take three long, smooth breaths. Concentrate on what you'd like your day-to-day life to be like. Then write statements as if those things have already occurred. For example: *I am grateful for living in an easily affordable house with all the space and amenities I desire.* Be as specific as you can vision.

I am grateful for _____

_____

I am grateful for _____

_____

I am grateful for _____

_____

I am grateful for _____

_____

I am grateful for _____

_____

I am grateful for _____

_____

I am grateful for _____

_____

I am grateful for _____

_____

GRATITUDE INTENTIONS FOR MY CAREER OR SCHOOL

Create statements about what you'd like to happen with your work or your studies. Then write as if those things have already occurred. For example: *I am grateful for having received the promotion and raise I've been working for.*

I am grateful for _____

_____

I am grateful for _____

_____

I am grateful for _____

_____

I am grateful for _____

_____

I am grateful for _____

_____

I am grateful for _____

_____

I am grateful for _____

_____

I am grateful for _____

_____

I am grateful for _____

_____

GRATITUDE INTENTIONS FOR MY FAMILY & MY RELATIONSHIPS WITH THEM

Create statements about what you'd like to happen for people you care deeply about. Then write as if those things have already occurred. For example: *I am grateful for my sister getting into the college of her dreams and my being able to support her.*

I am grateful for _____
_____

I am grateful for _____
_____

I am grateful for _____
_____

I am grateful for _____
_____

I am grateful for _____
_____

I am grateful for _____
_____

I am grateful for _____
_____

I am grateful for _____
_____

GRATITUDE INTENTIONS FOR PEOPLE I CONSIDER FAMILY

Create statements about what you'd like to happen for your family. Then write as if those things have already occurred. Some examples: *I am grateful for all of us being able to get together for my great grandfather's 90th birthday. I am grateful for my mom's new job.*

I am grateful for _____

_____

I am grateful for _____

_____

I am grateful for _____

_____

I am grateful for _____

_____

I am grateful for _____

_____

I am grateful for _____

_____

I am grateful for _____

_____

I am grateful for _____

_____

I am grateful for _____

_____

GRATITUDE INTENTIONS FOR MY FRIENDS & COMMUNITY

Create statements about what you'd like to happen for your friends and community members. Then write as if those things have already occurred. For example: *I am grateful for my friend Cathy's new business venture being financially successful now.*

I am grateful for _____

_____

I am grateful for _____

_____

I am grateful for _____

_____

I am grateful for _____

_____

I am grateful for _____

_____

I am grateful for _____

_____

I am grateful for _____

_____

I am grateful for _____

_____

GRATITUDE INTENTIONS FOR MY RELATIONSHIPS

Create statements about what you'd like to happen for your relationships. Then write as if those things have already occurred. For example: *I am grateful for finding a partner to travel with through life.*

I am grateful for _____
_____

I am grateful for _____
_____

I am grateful for _____
_____

I am grateful for _____
_____

I am grateful for _____
_____

I am grateful for _____
_____

I am grateful for _____
_____

I am grateful for _____
_____

GRATITUDE INTENTIONS FOR MY PROSPERITY & ABUNDANCE

Create statements about what you'd like to happen for yourself. Then write as if those things have already occurred. For example: *I am grateful for my excellent health and strong, fit body. I am grateful for living in a neighborhood I feel comfortable in.*

HEALTH & FITNESS

I am grateful for _____

I am grateful for _____

I am grateful for _____

I am grateful for _____

I am grateful for _____

WHERE I LIVE

I am grateful for _____

I am grateful for _____

I am grateful for _____

I am grateful for _____

I am grateful for _____

GRATITUDE INTENTIONS FOR MY PROSPERITY & ABUNDANCE

Create statements about what you'd like to happen for yourself. Then write as if those things have already occurred. For example: *I am grateful for my abundant financial prosperity that provides for all my needs and wants.*

MY FINANCES

I am grateful for _____

I am grateful for _____

I am grateful for _____

I am grateful for _____

I am grateful for _____

MY SAVINGS & PROPERTY

I am grateful for _____

I am grateful for _____

I am grateful for _____

I am grateful for _____

I am grateful for _____

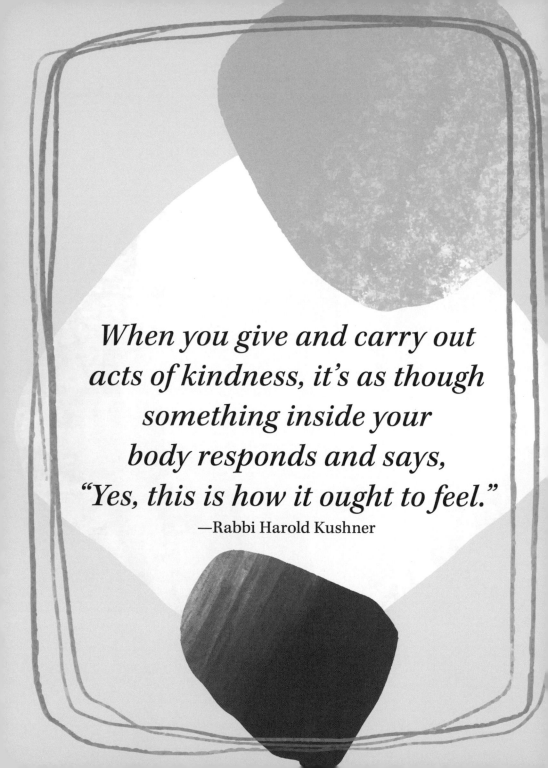

When you give and carry out
acts of kindness, it's as though
something inside your
body responds and says,
"Yes, this is how it ought to feel."
—Rabbi Harold Kushner

KINDNESS GRATITUDES

Experiencing the Value of Kindness

Kindness is a gift that can be easily given and received every day. It can be as simple as helping a stranger, checking in on a neighbor, or sending a quick text to a friend. Each of these efforts takes only a moment, but it has the power to change someone's day, including your own. Whether you are extending a hand or accepting a helping hand, warmth, happiness, and joy are always present. So, share yourself, and your kindness—you will feel the difference.

THE KINDNESS OF PEOPLE

Today, I am grateful that I was kind to these people.

I am grateful for _____

_____

I am grateful for _____

_____

I am grateful for _____

_____

I am grateful for _____

_____

I am grateful for _____

_____

Today, these people were kind to me.

I am grateful for _____

_____

I am grateful for _____

_____

I am grateful for _____

_____

I am grateful for _____

_____

I am grateful for _____

_____

DAILY PRACTICE

Fill in the blanks with people, things, and events you are grateful for today. On some days you might feel like adding more—do so. On the days when it is more difficult to fill in the blanks, remember that you can be grateful for everybody and anything.

DATE:

I am grateful for _____

I am grateful for _____

I am grateful for _____

I am grateful for _____

I am grateful for _____

FIVE GRATITUDE INTENTIONS

Fill in the blanks with things you'd like to create in your daily life.

I am grateful for _____

I am grateful for _____

I am grateful for _____

I am grateful for _____

I am grateful for _____

Today I feel gratitude in my _____

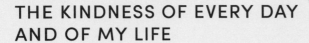

THE KINDNESS OF EVERY DAY
AND OF MY LIFE

These are simple everyday kindnesses that I received.

I am grateful for _____

_____

I am grateful for _____

_____

I am grateful for _____

_____

I am grateful for _____

_____

I am grateful for _____

_____

These are kindnesses that changed my life.

I am grateful for _____

_____

I am grateful for _____

_____

I am grateful for _____

_____

I am grateful for _____

_____

I am grateful for _____

_____

DAILY PRACTICE

Fill in the blanks with people, things, and events you are grateful for today. On some days you might feel like adding more—do so. On the days when it is more difficult to fill in the blanks, remember that you can be grateful for everybody and anything.

DATE: _____

I am grateful for _____

I am grateful for _____

I am grateful for _____

I am grateful for _____

I am grateful for _____

FIVE GRATITUDE INTENTIONS
Fill in the blanks with things you'd like to create in your daily life.

I am grateful for _____

I am grateful for _____

I am grateful for _____

I am grateful for _____

I am grateful for _____

Today I feel gratitude in my _____

THE KINDNESS OF LISTENING

Listening to someone so that they feel heard is a powerful and generous gift. It can assuage feelings of loneliness, isolation, and fear, to name a few. Below, express gratitude for conversations in which you were a trusted listener, and conversations in which you felt heard.

I am grateful I was able to listen to _____ when they talked about _____.

I am grateful I was able to listen to _____ when they talked about _____.

I am grateful I was able to listen to _____ when they talked about _____.

I am grateful I was able to listen to _____ when they talked about _____.

I am grateful _____ listened to me when I talked about _____.

I am grateful _____ listened to me when I talked about _____.

I am grateful _____ listened to me when I talked about _____.

I am grateful _____ listened to me when I talked about _____.

DAILY PRACTICE

Fill in the blanks with people, things, and events you are grateful for today. On some days you might feel like adding more—do so. On the days when it is more difficult to fill in the blanks, remember that you can be grateful for everybody and anything.

DATE: _____

I am grateful for _____

I am grateful for _____

I am grateful for _____

I am grateful for _____

I am grateful for _____

FIVE GRATITUDE INTENTIONS
Fill in the blanks with things you'd like to create in your daily life.

I am grateful for _____

I am grateful for _____

I am grateful for _____

I am grateful for _____

I am grateful for _____

Today I feel gratitude in my _____

THE KINDNESS OF CONNECTION

All of us need to feel connected to others. It helps our physical and mental well-being. A short "I am thinking of you" can positively shift someone's day as well as your own. List below people you have reached out to lately to let them know you care.

I am grateful for reaching out to _____

I am grateful for reaching out to _____

I am grateful for reaching out to _____

I am grateful for reaching out to _____

I am grateful for reaching out to _____

Now is a good time to reconnect with people who you've been thinking about but lost touch with. Fill in the gratitudes below with names of those you reconnected with or are thinking about reconnecting with.

I am grateful for reconnecting with

_____

I am grateful for reconnecting with

_____

I am grateful for reconnecting with

_____

I am grateful for reconnecting with

_____

I am grateful for reconnecting with

_____

DAILY PRACTICE

Fill in the blanks with people, things, and events you are grateful for today. On some days you might feel like adding more—do so. On the days when it is more difficult to fill in the blanks, remember that you can be grateful for everybody and anything.

DATE: _____

I am grateful for _____

I am grateful for _____

I am grateful for _____

I am grateful for _____

I am grateful for _____

FIVE GRATITUDE INTENTIONS
Fill in the blanks with things you'd like to create in your daily life.

I am grateful for _____

I am grateful for _____

I am grateful for _____

I am grateful for _____

I am grateful for _____

Today I feel gratitude in my _____

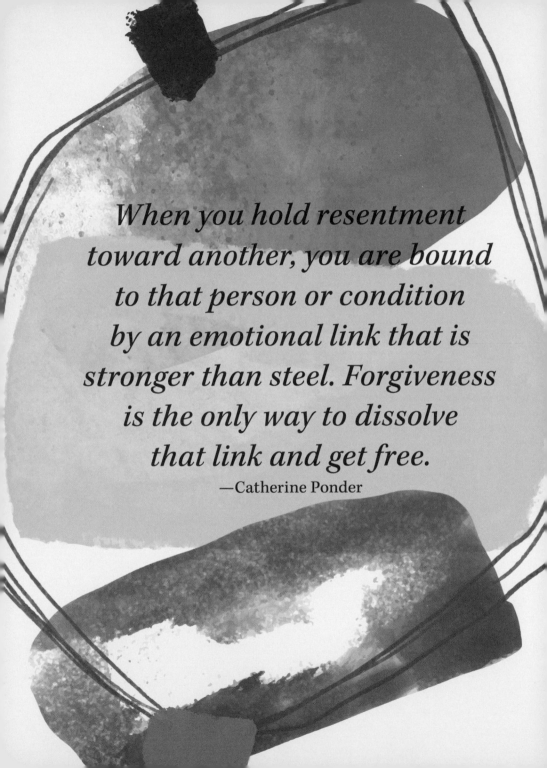

When you hold resentment toward another, you are bound to that person or condition by an emotional link that is stronger than steel. Forgiveness is the only way to dissolve that link and get free.

—Catherine Ponder

FORGIVENESS GRATITUDES

Giving the Gift of Forgiveness

Forgiveness is another one of those incredibly simple and powerful tools. It is a gift to each and every one of us. It gives us the freedom to move forward unencumbered. Whether we are forgiving ourselves or someone else, forgiveness allows us to let go of the hurt, anger, and upset, and to heal. Forgiving someone does not excuse the transgression; however, it frees us to heal and move on. As we master the art of forgiveness, we will find ourselves less burdened by the small and large upsets of life. Being able to forgive also helps us build resilience. Forgiveness is not always easy, but with practice it can become so.

SELF-FORGIVENESS

We need to learn to forgive ourselves for things we regret doing. Here is a safe place to release your regrets and forgive yourself for the things you wish you hadn't done. In learning to forgive ourselves, we also learn to be more forgiving of others.

I gratefully forgive myself for

_____

I gratefully forgive myself for

_____

I gratefully forgive myself for

_____

I gratefully forgive myself for

_____

I gratefully forgive myself for

_____

I gratefully forgive myself for

_____

I gratefully forgive myself for

_____

I gratefully forgive myself for

_____

I gratefully forgive myself for

_____

I gratefully forgive myself for

_____

DAILY PRACTICE

Fill in the blanks with people, things, and events you are grateful for today. On some days you might feel like adding more—do so. On the days when it is more difficult to fill in the blanks, remember that you can be grateful for everybody and anything.

DATE:

I am grateful for _____

I am grateful for _____

I am grateful for _____

I am grateful for _____

I am grateful for _____

FIVE GRATITUDE INTENTIONS
Fill in the blanks with things you'd like to create in your daily life.

I am grateful for _____

I am grateful for _____

I am grateful for _____

I am grateful for _____

I am grateful for _____

Today I feel gratitude in my _____

FORGIVENESS OF OTHERS

Use the gratitudes below to forgive those who have hurt you. Remember this is a gift to yourself—to let go of all the anger, hurt, betrayal, and other negative feelings. "I forgive you" means *I release myself from the harm you caused.* This is a private page just for you. If you want, you can share your forgiveness thoughts and statements with those you forgive. It is up to you.

I am grateful for forgiving

_____

I am grateful for forgiving

_____

I am grateful for forgiving

_____

I am grateful for forgiving

_____

I am grateful for forgiving

_____

I am grateful for forgiving

_____

I am grateful for forgiving

_____

I am grateful for forgiving

_____

I am grateful for forgiving

_____

I am grateful for forgiving

_____

DAILY PRACTICE

Fill in the blanks with people, things, and events you are grateful for today. On some days you might feel like adding more—do so. On the days when it is more difficult to fill in the blanks, remember that you can be grateful for everybody and anything.

DATE:

I am grateful for _____

I am grateful for _____

I am grateful for _____

I am grateful for _____

I am grateful for _____

FIVE GRATITUDE INTENTIONS
Fill in the blanks with things you'd like to create in your daily life.

I am grateful for _____

I am grateful for _____

I am grateful for _____

I am grateful for _____

I am grateful for _____

Today I feel gratitude in my _____

LETTING GO WITH FORGIVENESS

Fill this page with experiences that you are grateful to let go of.

I am grateful for letting go of

_____

I am grateful for letting go of

_____

I am grateful for letting go of

_____

I am grateful for letting go of

_____

I am grateful for letting go of

_____

I am grateful for letting go of

_____

I am grateful for letting go of

_____

I am grateful for letting go of

_____

I am grateful for letting go of

_____

I am grateful for letting go of

_____

DAILY PRACTICE

Fill in the blanks with people, things, and events you are grateful for today. On some days you might feel like adding more—do so. On the days when it is more difficult to fill in the blanks, remember that you can be grateful for everybody and anything.

DATE:

I am grateful for _____

I am grateful for _____

I am grateful for _____

I am grateful for _____

I am grateful for _____

FIVE GRATITUDE INTENTIONS
Fill in the blanks with things you'd like to create in your daily life.

I am grateful for _____

I am grateful for _____

I am grateful for _____

I am grateful for _____

I am grateful for _____

Today I feel gratitude in my _____

FORGIVE ME

This page is for you to recognize any people you'd like to forgive you. It can be for a significant transgression or an innocent mistake. This exercise is just for you, so open your heart and allow it to heal.

I am grateful for _____ forgiving me.

I am grateful for _____ forgiving me.

I am grateful for _____ forgiving me.

I am grateful for _____ forgiving me.

I am grateful for _____ forgiving me.

I am grateful for _____ forgiving me.

I am grateful for _____ forgiving me.

I am grateful for _____ forgiving me.

I am grateful for _____ forgiving me.

I am grateful for _____ forgiving me.

DAILY PRACTICE

Fill in the blanks with people, things, and events you are grateful for today. On some days you might feel like adding more—do so. On the days when it is more difficult to fill in the blanks, remember that you can be grateful for everybody and anything.

DATE:

I am grateful for _____

I am grateful for _____

I am grateful for _____

I am grateful for _____

I am grateful for _____

FIVE GRATITUDE INTENTIONS
Fill in the blanks with things you'd like to create in your daily life.

I am grateful for _____

I am grateful for _____

I am grateful for _____

I am grateful for _____

I am grateful for _____

Today I feel gratitude in my _____

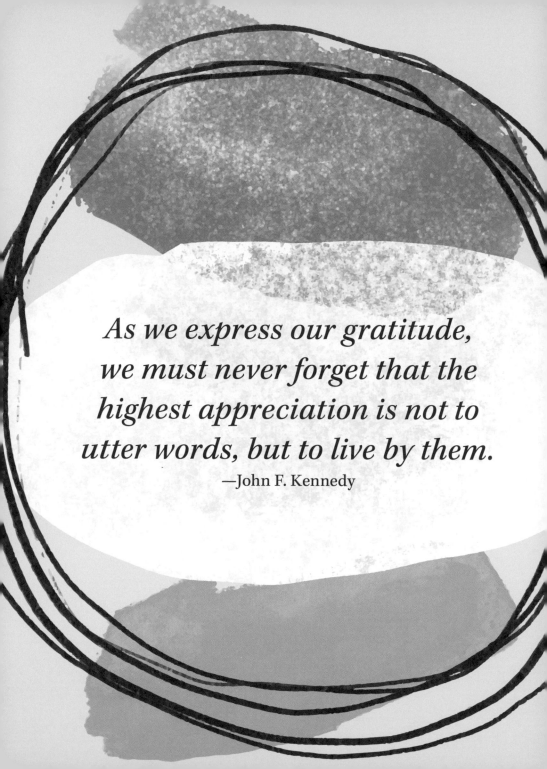

As we express our gratitude, we must never forget that the highest appreciation is not to utter words, but to live by them.

—John F. Kennedy

BEING OF SERVICE GRATITUDES

Taking Care of Yourself and Others

Helping others and assisting in something that is bigger than ourselves can provide purpose in our lives. Research suggests that being of service helps the mind and body heal. Recognizing your service and expressing gratitude for it can positively affect how we feel emotionally, mentally, and even physically. When we give to others from the heart, we receive as much in return. Unexpected joy will break through even during the most challenging times to keep us going.

HELPING & ASSISTING OTHERS

Acknowledge how you helped someone in a way that made you feel good. For example: *I am grateful for helping families with purchasing groceries when they needed food.*

I am grateful for helping _____
with _____

I am grateful for helping _____
with _____

I am grateful for helping _____
with _____

I am grateful for helping _____
with _____

Record actions and things you were grateful to provide for an organization or group. For example: *I am grateful for assisting the school with getting additional supplies.*

I am grateful for assisting _____
with _____

I am grateful for assisting _____
with _____

I am grateful for assisting _____
with _____

I am grateful for assisting _____
with _____

DAILY PRACTICE

Fill in the blanks with people, things, and events you are grateful for today. On some days you might feel like adding more—do so. On the days when it is more difficult to fill in the blanks, remember that you can be grateful for everybody and anything.

DATE: _____

I am grateful for _____

I am grateful for _____

I am grateful for _____

I am grateful for _____

I am grateful for _____

FIVE GRATITUDE INTENTIONS
Fill in the blanks with things you'd like to create in your daily life.

I am grateful for _____

I am grateful for _____

I am grateful for _____

I am grateful for _____

I am grateful for _____

Today I feel gratitude in my _____

SHOWING I CARE

Write about all those caring, beautiful things you regularly do for others that make a difference in their lives. Some examples: *I am grateful for making a difference for my family by cooking dinner many nights a week. I am grateful for making a difference for my friends by making them laugh with my jokes.*

I am grateful for making a difference for

_____

by _____

I am grateful for making a difference for

_____

by _____

I am grateful for making a difference for

_____

by _____

I am grateful for making a difference for

_____

by _____

I am grateful for making a difference for

_____

by _____

I am grateful for making a difference for

_____

by _____

I am grateful for making a difference for

_____

by _____

DAILY PRACTICE

Fill in the blanks with people, things, and events you are grateful for today. On some days you might feel like adding more—do so. On the days when it is more difficult to fill in the blanks, remember that you can be grateful for everybody and anything.

DATE: _____

I am grateful for _____

I am grateful for _____

I am grateful for _____

I am grateful for _____

I am grateful for _____

FIVE GRATITUDE INTENTIONS
Fill in the blanks with things you'd like to create in your daily life.

I am grateful for _____

I am grateful for _____

I am grateful for _____

I am grateful for _____

I am grateful for _____

Today I feel gratitude in my _____

MAKING CONTRIBUTIONS

Every day we make contributions to others, and most often we don't even recognize it. Spend some time considering what you do for others. Use the space below to acknowledge and be grateful for the many things you do for others. You can include everything from giving monetary donations to helping specific organizations, giving your time, listening to a friend, shoveling snow for a neighbor, and more.

I am grateful for contributing to _____

I am grateful for contributing to _____

I am grateful for contributing to _____

I am grateful for contributing to _____

I am grateful for contributing to _____

I am grateful for contributing to _____

I am grateful for contributing to _____

I am grateful for contributing to _____

I am grateful for contributing to _____

I am grateful for contributing to _____

DAILY PRACTICE

Fill in the blanks with people, things, and events you are grateful for today. On some days you might feel like adding more—do so. On the days when it is more difficult to fill in the blanks, remember that you can be grateful for everybody and anything.

DATE:

I am grateful for _____

I am grateful for _____

I am grateful for _____

I am grateful for _____

I am grateful for _____

FIVE GRATITUDE INTENTIONS
Fill in the blanks with things you'd like to create in your daily life.

I am grateful for _____

I am grateful for _____

I am grateful for _____

I am grateful for _____

I am grateful for _____

Today I feel gratitude in my _____

VOLUNTEERING

Some projects and issues take a larger group of people to make things happen. Here, you can express your gratitude for participating in the following community groups and organizations to make a difference.

I am grateful for being a member of _____ _____ and doing work to help _____

I am grateful for being a member of _____ _____ and doing work to help _____

I am grateful for being a member of _____ _____ and doing work to help _____

I am grateful for participating with _____ _____ to contribute to _____

I am grateful for participating with _____ _____ to contribute to _____

I am grateful for participating with _____ _____ to contribute to _____

DAILY PRACTICE

Fill in the blanks with people, things, and events you are grateful for today. On some days you might feel like adding more—do so. On the days when it is more difficult to fill in the blanks, remember that you can be grateful for everybody and anything.

DATE:

I am grateful for _____

I am grateful for _____

I am grateful for _____

I am grateful for _____

I am grateful for _____

FIVE GRATITUDE INTENTIONS
Fill in the blanks with things you'd like to create in your daily life.

I am grateful for _____

I am grateful for _____

I am grateful for _____

I am grateful for _____

I am grateful for _____

Today I feel gratitude in my _____

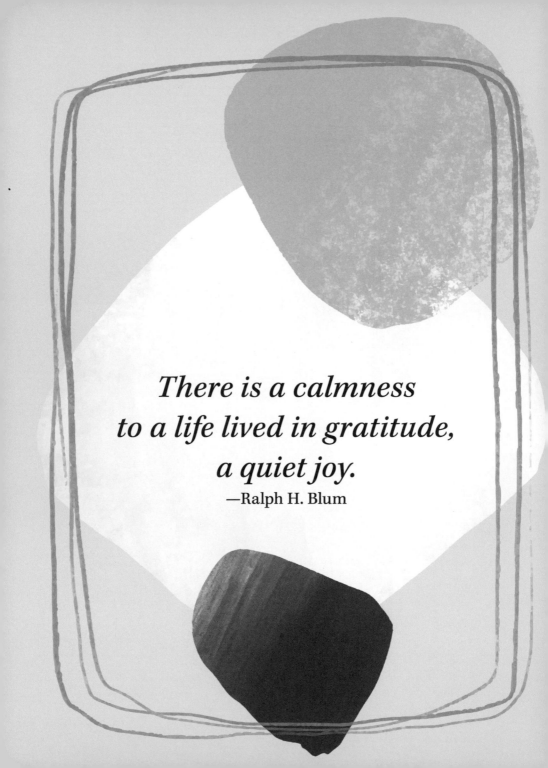

*There is a calmness
to a life lived in gratitude,
a quiet joy.*

—Ralph H. Blum

QUIET GRATITUDE MOMENTS

Experiencing Gratitude

In this world that is moving faster than ever with constant distractions vying for our attention, many of us have forgotten how to embrace the quiet. To sit serenely and watch a sunset. To meditate or pray before we rise. To savor our food as we eat a meal. To listen to our favorite music, or to engage with a piece of artwork. Most of us need to relearn this skill as we are out of practice. This section uses gratitude and gratitude statements to guide you in learning to be still and to be present.

TAKE A MOMENT TO NOTICE

It is through being grateful that we can find comfort, happiness, and contentment even during challenging times to appreciate and be here now. Write the moments you notice that you are grateful for. For example: *Today, I am grateful for noticing the brilliant colors of the sunset.*

Today, I am grateful for noticing

_____

Today, I am grateful for noticing

_____

Today, I am grateful for noticing

_____

Today, I am grateful for noticing

_____

Today, I am grateful for noticing

_____

Today, I am grateful for noticing

_____

Today, I am grateful for noticing

_____

Today, I am grateful for noticing

_____

Today, I am grateful for noticing

_____

Today, I am grateful for noticing

_____

DAILY PRACTICE

Fill in the blanks with people, things, and events you are grateful for today. On some days you might feel like adding more—do so. On the days when it is more difficult to fill in the blanks, remember that you can be grateful for everybody and anything.

DATE:

I am grateful for _____

I am grateful for _____

I am grateful for _____

I am grateful for _____

I am grateful for _____

FIVE GRATITUDE INTENTIONS
Fill in the blanks with things you'd like to create in your daily life.

I am grateful for _____

I am grateful for _____

I am grateful for _____

I am grateful for _____

I am grateful for _____

Today I feel gratitude in my _____

TAKE A MOMENT TO BE THANKFUL

Make it part of your day to pause, watch, and observe what is going on around you. Express gratitude for those happenings that make you think, smile, and laugh.

Today, I am grateful for watching

_____

Today, I am grateful for watching

_____

Today, I am grateful for watching

_____

Today, I am grateful for watching

_____

Today, I am grateful for watching

_____

Today, I am grateful for watching

_____

Today, I am grateful for watching

_____

Today, I am grateful for watching

_____

Today, I am grateful for watching

_____

Today, I am grateful for watching

_____

DAILY PRACTICE

Fill in the blanks with people, things, and events you are grateful for today. On some days you might feel like adding more—do so. On the days when it is more difficult to fill in the blanks, remember that you can be grateful for everybody and anything.

DATE:

I am grateful for _____

I am grateful for _____

I am grateful for _____

I am grateful for _____

I am grateful for _____

FIVE GRATITUDE INTENTIONS
Fill in the blanks with things you'd like to create in your daily life.

I am grateful for _____

I am grateful for _____

I am grateful for _____

I am grateful for _____

I am grateful for _____

Today I feel gratitude in my _____

TAKE A MOMENT TO ACCEPT

This one can be difficult to do, but when mastered it provides much comfort. Acceptance does not mean resignation. It means to be in the moment, accept how it is, and allow yourself to create solutions without falling into anger, depression, or despair. That is why you might hear people who have learned acceptance say things like, "My illness was a gift. I learned so much from my recovery." Fill in the gratitude statements below with things from your life that you found particularly hard.

I am grateful for accepting

_____

I am grateful for accepting

_____

I am grateful for accepting

_____

I am grateful for accepting

_____

I am grateful for accepting

_____

DAILY PRACTICE

Fill in the blanks with people, things, and events you are grateful for today. On some days you might feel like adding more—do so. On the days when it is more difficult to fill in the blanks, remember that you can be grateful for everybody and anything.

DATE:

I am grateful for _____

I am grateful for _____

I am grateful for _____

I am grateful for _____

I am grateful for _____

FIVE GRATITUDE INTENTIONS
Fill in the blanks with things you'd like to create in your daily life.

I am grateful for _____

I am grateful for _____

I am grateful for _____

I am grateful for _____

I am grateful for _____

Today I feel gratitude in my _____

TAKE A MOMENT TO THINK

Here is your space to capture thoughts that cause you to pause, think, and consider. It can be ideas for the future, memories from the past, or contemplations of the present.

I am grateful for thinking about

_____

_____

I am grateful for thinking about

_____

_____

I am grateful for thinking about

_____

_____

I am grateful for thinking about

_____

_____

I am grateful for thinking about

_____

_____

DAILY PRACTICE

Fill in the blanks with people, things, and events you are grateful for today. On some days you might feel like adding more—do so. On the days when it is more difficult to fill in the blanks, remember that you can be grateful for everybody and anything.

DATE:

I am grateful for _____

I am grateful for _____

I am grateful for _____

I am grateful for _____

I am grateful for _____

FIVE GRATITUDE INTENTIONS
Fill in the blanks with things you'd like to create in your daily life.

I am grateful for _____

I am grateful for _____

I am grateful for _____

I am grateful for _____

I am grateful for _____

Today I feel gratitude in my _____

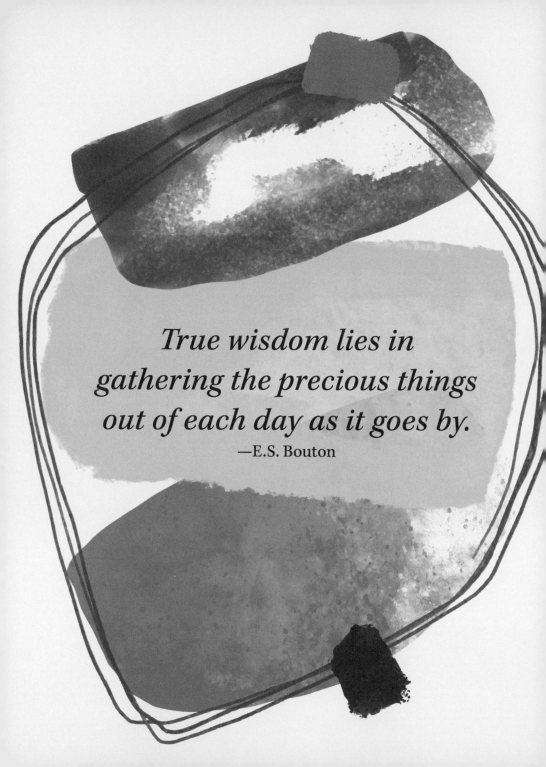

True wisdom lies in gathering the precious things out of each day as it goes by.

—E.S. Bouton

GRATITUDE MEDITATIONS

Cultivating Gratitude

Developing a meditation practice can be life affirming. There are many approaches to meditation, but here is a short, accessible gratitude meditation for you to engage.

First, find a comfortable place to lie down or to sit upright. Once you're situated, set a timer for five minutes. Close your eyes. Notice your breath. Observe your breathing for five inhalations and five exhalations.

Now picture in your mind's eye a beautiful, serene, and quiet place. A place you feel safe and protected. A place you feel grateful to be enjoying. Settle into that space and allow your breath to flow.

Choose one person, place, or thing you are grateful for to focus on. It is okay if you find your mind wanders. When you notice that happening, just bring your focus back to your gratitude choice.

When your timer goes off, gently open your eyes. Take a few minutes to reorient to your current space. Slowly rise.

BREATH WORK

Breathing is such a natural thing. For the most part, it just happens without us having to think about it. However, learning to observe and control your breath is a useful skill. It can help keep you calm when facing challenges, upsets, anxiety, or fear.

To begin, sit or lie in a comfortable position. Set a timer for five minutes or more. Close your eyes. Then close your mouth and breathe through your nose. Notice your breath. Are your inhalations deep or shallow? Are the exhalations the same quality as the inhalations? Keep the breath moving freely, steadily and easily, until the timer goes off. Capture what you observed and experienced below.

I am grateful for noticing my breath was

_____

I am grateful for noticing my breath was

_____

I am grateful for noticing my breath was

_____

I am grateful during the exercise for feeling

_____

I am grateful during the exercise for feeling

_____

I am grateful during the exercise for feeling

_____

DAILY PRACTICE

Fill in the blanks with people, things, and events you are grateful for today. On some days you might feel like adding more—do so. On the days when it is more difficult to fill in the blanks, remember that you can be grateful for everybody and anything.

DATE:

I am grateful for _____

I am grateful for _____

I am grateful for _____

I am grateful for _____

I am grateful for _____

FIVE GRATITUDE INTENTIONS
Fill in the blanks with things you'd like to create in your daily life.

I am grateful for _____

I am grateful for _____

I am grateful for _____

I am grateful for _____

I am grateful for _____

Today I feel gratitude in my _____

GRATITUDE WALK

Staying physically active and moving everyday helps us stay healthy. The Gratitude Walk combines the physical need for movement with the whole body's desire for happiness. Your walk can be the length that works best for you. Select a route in which you can safely move at your pace and say gratitudes out loud or in your mind. Say at least ten gratitudes, but don't let that number limit you. They can all be inspired by your walking experience or from other aspects of your life.

When you return, write down as many gratitude statements as you like and take a picture of them with your phone so they're handy to read in moments of frustration, anger, and upset. You will find that saying, reading, and writing gratitude statements will help calm the mind and body.

I am grateful for _____

I am grateful for _____

I am grateful for _____

I am grateful for _____

I am grateful for _____

I am grateful for _____

I am grateful for _____

I am grateful for _____

I am grateful for _____

I am grateful for _____

DAILY PRACTICE

Fill in the blanks with people, things, and events you are grateful for today. On some days you might feel like adding more—do so. On the days when it is more difficult to fill in the blanks, remember that you can be grateful for everybody and anything.

DATE:

I am grateful for _____

I am grateful for _____

I am grateful for _____

I am grateful for _____

I am grateful for _____

FIVE GRATITUDE INTENTIONS
Fill in the blanks with things you'd like to create in your daily life.

I am grateful for _____

I am grateful for _____

I am grateful for _____

I am grateful for _____

I am grateful for _____

Today I feel gratitude in my _____

GRATITUDE HIKE

This is for days when you have time to get away and be outdoors. Select a hiking path that is surrounded by nature. Choose a route that works for your body. If possible, spend an hour or more walking with occasional stops to write a couple of gratitude statements. Commit to having at least ten gratitude statements written when you complete your hike, but don't let that number limit you. Write your statements in the space below. Begin each statement with "I am grateful for."

-
-
-
-
-
-
-
-
-
-

DAILY PRACTICE

Fill in the blanks with people, things, and events you are grateful for today. On some days you might feel like adding more—do so. On the days when it is more difficult to fill in the blanks, remember that you can be grateful for everybody and anything.

DATE:

I am grateful for _____

I am grateful for _____

I am grateful for _____

I am grateful for _____

I am grateful for _____

FIVE GRATITUDE INTENTIONS
Fill in the blanks with things you'd like to create in your daily life.

I am grateful for _____

I am grateful for _____

I am grateful for _____

I am grateful for _____

I am grateful for _____

Today I feel gratitude in my _____

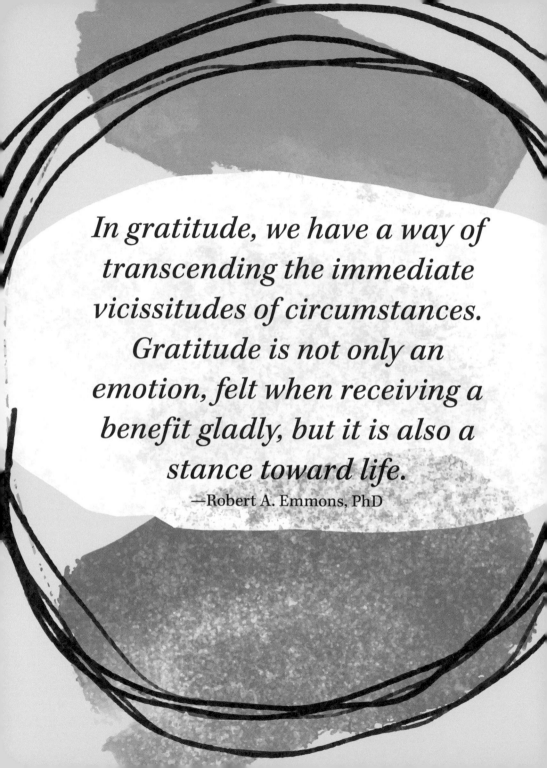

In gratitude, we have a way of transcending the immediate vicissitudes of circumstances. Gratitude is not only an emotion, felt when receiving a benefit gladly, but it is also a stance toward life.

—Robert A. Emmons, PhD

GRATITUDES FOR THE HARD DAYS
Using Gratitude During Difficult Times

Some days are just hard. The challenges from life seem heavy. On these days, thinking about generating gratitude statements may feel impossible. This section is for those days. It is not to be used as an excuse to avoid creating one's own gratitudes, but to be used when everything feels overwhelmingly difficult.

GRATITUDE STATEMENTS FOR THE CHALLENGING DAYS

When you are feeling upset, overwhelmed, angry, hurt, betrayed, or any type of pain, you can reach for this list to read and reread.

- I am grateful for today.
- I am grateful for all the beauty in the world.
- I am grateful for the sunrise.
- I am grateful for a gorgeous sky.
- I am grateful for fresh air.
- I am grateful for a warm breeze.
- I am grateful for a sunny day.
- I am grateful for time outdoors.
- I am grateful for peaceful moments.
- I am grateful for genuine caring.

- I am grateful for seeing the positive.
- I am grateful for abundance.
- I am grateful for all acts of kindness.
- I am grateful for being able to help others.
- I am grateful for keeping my cool today.
- I am grateful for those who support me.
- I am grateful for the smiles I receive.
- I am grateful for a gentle hug.
- I am grateful for today's opportunities.
- I am grateful for forgiving and being forgiven.

DAILY PRACTICE

For your daily practice, read the gratitude statements below. If you can push yourself at all, feel free to add your own in the margins. Having gratitude statements to read on the really difficult days helps you keep your gratitude practice going. You can use the statements below or from any page in the journal.

GRATITUDES FOR TODAY
I am grateful for my determination.
I am grateful for my friends and family.
I am grateful for my health and vitality.
I am grateful for having faith in myself.
I am grateful for being me.

GRATITUDE INTENTIONS FOR TODAY
I am grateful for my abundant financial prosperity.
I am grateful for my resilience that allows me to
*   bounce back from adversity.*
I am grateful for my hopes and dreams
*   manifesting now.*
I am grateful for my courage to reach
*   for the stars.*
I am grateful for having the strength
*   to never give up.*

Identify on the outline where you feel the gratitude today.

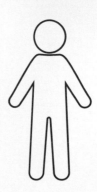

PERSONAL GRATITUDE STATEMENTS

These statements are more personal. They reflect positive feelings you have or would like to have about yourself. Research reveals that our thoughts affect our well-being, so read the statements below, either out loud or silently. Repeating these statements helps especially on the hard days to create new plasticity and build your resilience.

- I am grateful, for I am loved.
- I am grateful for finding peace.
- I am grateful for loving myself as I am.
- I am grateful for accepting myself.
- I am grateful for forgiving myself.
- I am grateful for releasing my fears
- I am grateful, for I am heard and respected.
- I am grateful for giving to and receiving from my community.
- I am grateful to smile every day.
- I am grateful for new, engaging experiences.

DAILY PRACTICE

For your daily practice, read the gratitude statements below. If you can push yourself at all, feel free to add your own in the margins. Having gratitude statements to read on the really difficult days helps you keep your gratitude practice going. You can use the statements below or from any page in the journal.

GRATITUDES FOR TODAY
I am grateful for my determination.
I am grateful for my friends and family.
I am grateful for my health and vitality.
I am grateful for having faith in myself.
I am grateful for being me.

GRATITUDE INTENTIONS FOR TODAY
I am grateful for my abundant financial prosperity.
I am grateful for my resilience that allows me to
* bounce back from adversity.*
I am grateful for my hopes and dreams
* manifesting now.*
I am grateful for my courage to reach
* for the stars.*
I am grateful for having the strength
* to never give up.*

Identify on the outline where you feel the gratitude today.

I AM GRATEFUL FOR DOING THINGS TO HELP MYSELF

When we are feeling distraught, depressed, or generally down, the activities on this page will help you pick yourself up, dust yourself off, and start all over again. Choose one of the activities and do it. Then fill in the gratitude statement about what you have accomplished.

CREATE SOMETHING—ANYTHING. Sing a song, make a favorite snack or food, paint, color, write, or send a humorous text. It is the act of creating something that did not exist before that helps you to feel better.

I am grateful for making

_____

PLAY, BE SILLY, OR DO BOTH! Allow that childlike enthusiasm to surface and guide you to doing something just to do it. Something you enjoy that brings a smile, laughter, and even joy. Go ahead and let yourself loose—no one is watching.

I am grateful for _____

HELP SOMEONE TODAY. It is remarkable how helping someone gives us so much in return.

I am grateful for _____

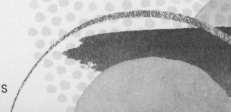

DAILY PRACTICE

For your daily practice, read the gratitude statements below. If you can push yourself at all, feel free to add your own in the margins. Having gratitude statements to read on the really difficult days helps you keep your gratitude practice going. You can use the statements below or from any page in the journal.

GRATITUDES FOR TODAY
I am grateful for my determination.
I am grateful for my friends and family.
I am grateful for my health and vitality.
I am grateful for having faith in myself.
I am grateful for being me.

GRATITUDE INTENTIONS FOR TODAY
I am grateful for my abundant financial prosperity.
I am grateful for my resilience that allows me to
   bounce back from adversity.
I am grateful for my hopes and dreams
   manifesting now.
I am grateful for my courage to reach
   for the stars.
I am grateful for having the strength
   to never give up.

Identify on the outline where you feel the gratitude today.

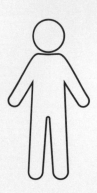

THE POWER OF SMILING & LAUGHTER

It is amazing how healing a smile, a chuckle, and a good laugh can be in the moment and over time. When you learn to laugh as a favorite tool, it opens doors to happiness when they previously felt closed by pain or fear. So sometimes you just have to focus on having a laugh. Fill in the statements with things you do now to smile and laugh, or memories that still make you happy.

I am grateful for _____ making me smile.
I am grateful for _____ making me smile.

I am grateful for chuckling over _____
I am grateful for chuckling over _____

I am grateful for laughing when

_____

I am grateful for laughing when

_____

I am grateful for laughing so hard when

_____

I am grateful for laughing so hard when

_____

DAILY PRACTICE

For your daily practice, read the gratitude statements below. If you can push yourself at all, feel free to add your own in the margins. Having gratitude statements to read on the really difficult days helps you keep your gratitude practice going. You can use the statements below or from any page in the journal.

GRATITUDES FOR TODAY
I am grateful for my determination.
I am grateful for my friends and family.
I am grateful for my health and vitality.
I am grateful for having faith in myself.
I am grateful for being me.

GRATITUDE INTENTIONS FOR TODAY
I am grateful for my abundant financial prosperity.
I am grateful for my resilience that allows me to
bounce back from adversity.
I am grateful for my hopes and dreams
manifesting now.
I am grateful for my courage to reach
for the stars.
I am grateful for having the strength
to never give up.

Identify on the outline where you feel the gratitude today.

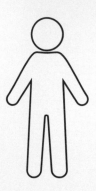

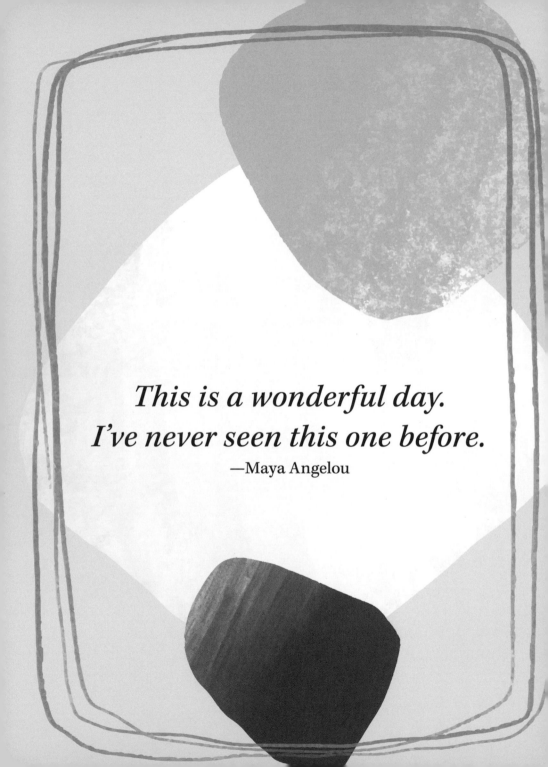

This is a wonderful day.
I've never seen this one before.

—Maya Angelou

GRATITUDES FOR THE FUTURE

Visioning the Life You Desire

This section is about creating the future you want. New discoveries in neuroscience are uncovering the importance of our thoughts and how they trigger physical, emotional, and psychological responses in our minds and bodies. So, close your eyes and think about what you will be doing one year from now... five years from now... and ten years from now. If you can see it, you can work to make it happen! Use your gratitude intentions to help you create a detailed picture of your vision.

MY FUTURE JOB AND CAREER

Fill in the gratitude statements with specifics about your dream job and career as if you already have it. For example: *I am grateful for being an entrepreneur owning 100% of my business.*

I am grateful for _____

I am grateful for _____

I am grateful for _____

I am grateful for _____

I am grateful for _____

I am grateful for _____

I am grateful for _____

I am grateful for _____

I am grateful for _____

I am grateful for _____

DAILY PRACTICE

Fill in the blanks with people, things, and events you are grateful for today. On some days you might feel like adding more—do so. On the days when it is more difficult to fill in the blanks, remember that you can be grateful for everybody and anything.

DATE:

I am grateful for _____

I am grateful for _____

I am grateful for _____

I am grateful for _____

I am grateful for _____

FIVE GRATITUDE INTENTIONS

Fill in the blanks with things you'd like to create in your daily life.

I am grateful for _____

I am grateful for _____

I am grateful for _____

I am grateful for _____

I am grateful for _____

Today I feel gratitude in my _____

MY FUTURE FAMILY

Chronicle who you want your family to be comprised of, including friends and pets.

I am grateful for _____

I am grateful for _____

I am grateful for _____

I am grateful for _____

I am grateful for _____

I am grateful for _____

I am grateful for _____

I am grateful for _____

Describe who your most important relationships are with and what they look like.

I am grateful for _____

I am grateful for _____

I am grateful for _____

I am grateful for _____

I am grateful for _____

I am grateful for _____

I am grateful for _____

I am grateful for _____

DAILY PRACTICE

Fill in the blanks with people, things, and events you are grateful for today. On some days you might feel like adding more—do so. On the days when it is more difficult to fill in the blanks, remember that you can be grateful for everybody and anything.

DATE:

I am grateful for _____

I am grateful for _____

I am grateful for _____

I am grateful for _____

I am grateful for _____

FIVE GRATITUDE INTENTIONS
Fill in the blanks with things you'd like to create in your daily life.

I am grateful for _____

I am grateful for _____

I am grateful for _____

I am grateful for _____

I am grateful for _____

Today I feel gratitude in my _____

MY FUTURE LIFE

Detail the lifestyle you would like to live and write as if you already have it. Some examples: *I am grateful for being able to travel when I want to. I am grateful for my own home. I am grateful for having season tickets for my favorite sports team. I am grateful for having time to volunteer at the local senior center. I am grateful for pursuing my goal to learn to play an instrument.*

I am grateful for _____

I am grateful for _____

I am grateful for _____

I am grateful for _____

I am grateful for _____

I am grateful for _____

I am grateful for _____

I am grateful for _____

I am grateful for _____

I am grateful for _____

I am grateful for _____

I am grateful for _____

I am grateful for _____

I am grateful for _____

I am grateful for _____

DAILY PRACTICE

Fill in the blanks with people, things, and events you are grateful for today. On some days you might feel like adding more—do so. On the days when it is more difficult to fill in the blanks, remember that you can be grateful for everybody and anything.

DATE:

I am grateful for _____

I am grateful for _____

I am grateful for _____

I am grateful for _____

I am grateful for _____

FIVE GRATITUDE INTENTIONS
Fill in the blanks with things you'd like to create in your daily life.

I am grateful for _____

I am grateful for _____

I am grateful for _____

I am grateful for _____

I am grateful for _____

Today I feel gratitude in my _____

GRATITUDES FOR MY FUTURE

On this page, envision what you'd like your life to look like over the next year, five years, and ten years. Create gratitude intention statements that reflect your visions.

In One Year from Now...

I am grateful for _____

I am grateful for _____

I am grateful for _____

I am grateful for _____

In Five Years from Now...

I am grateful for _____

I am grateful for _____

I am grateful for _____

I am grateful for _____

In Ten Years from Now...

I am grateful for _____

I am grateful for _____

I am grateful for _____

I am grateful for _____

DAILY PRACTICE

Fill in the blanks with people, things, and events you are grateful for today. On some days you might feel like adding more—do so. On the days when it is more difficult to fill in the blanks, remember that you can be grateful for everybody and anything.

DATE:

I am grateful for _____

I am grateful for _____

I am grateful for _____

I am grateful for _____

I am grateful for _____

FIVE GRATITUDE INTENTIONS
Fill in the blanks with things you'd like to create in your daily life.

I am grateful for _____

I am grateful for _____

I am grateful for _____

I am grateful for _____

I am grateful for _____

Today I feel gratitude in my _____

Follow your bliss and the universe will open doors where there were only walls.

—Joseph Campbell

PRIVATE THOUGHTS

Reflecting on Your Gratitudes

In these final pages, capture your learnings, experiences, thoughts, and feelings. Make sure to write down your insights and identify which practices work best for you. Record how you have or are going to incorporate gratitude tools in your life.

MY THOUGHTS & REFLECTIONS

Take some quiet time to think about your experience with gratitude and capture those thoughts on this page.

I'm feeling:

_____

_____

_____

I've been thinking about:

_____

_____

_____

I've noticed:

_____

_____

_____

Changes I'm considering are:

_____

_____

_____

DAILY PRACTICE

Fill in the blanks with people, things, and events you are grateful for today. On some days you might feel like adding more—do so. On the days when it is more difficult to fill in the blanks, remember that you can be grateful for everybody and anything.

DATE:

I am grateful for _____

I am grateful for _____

I am grateful for _____

I am grateful for _____

I am grateful for _____

FIVE GRATITUDE INTENTIONS
Fill in the blanks with things you'd like to create in your daily life.

I am grateful for _____

I am grateful for _____

I am grateful for _____

I am grateful for _____

I am grateful for _____

Today I feel gratitude in my _____

APPRECIATION STATEMENTS

Appreciation statements are ways to show our gratitude to those around us. There is never too much giving and receiving of kindness. However, in the busyness of daily life, we often forget to tell those we care about how much they mean to us. Below are appreciation statements for you to use on a daily basis, as well as space to create some of your own.

- I appreciate you.
- I appreciate all you do for me.
- I appreciate your support.
- I appreciate your kindness.
- I appreciate your generosity.
- I appreciate your patience.
- I appreciate your sense of humor.
- I appreciate your love.

I appreciate _____

I appreciate _____

I appreciate _____

I appreciate _____

I appreciate _____

I appreciate _____

I appreciate _____

DAILY PRACTICE

Fill in the blanks with people, things, and events you are grateful for today. On some days you might feel like adding more—do so. On the days when it is more difficult to fill in the blanks, remember that you can be grateful for everybody and anything.

DATE:

I am grateful for _____

I am grateful for _____

I am grateful for _____

I am grateful for _____

I am grateful for _____

FIVE GRATITUDE INTENTIONS
Fill in the blanks with things you'd like to create in your daily life.

I am grateful for _____

I am grateful for _____

I am grateful for _____

I am grateful for _____

I am grateful for _____

Today I feel gratitude in my _____

SPECIAL THANK-YOUS FOR MY LOVED ONES

Use the statements below or create personalized statements to express your gratitude to your loved ones. Fill in the blanks with names and your personal thank-you to each person.

- Thank you for being there for me.
- Thank you for believing in me.
- Thank you for doing everything you do.
- Thank you for caring enough about me to say no.
- Thank you for trusting me.
- Thank you being you.
- Thank you for loving me just the way I am.
- Thank you for making me laugh.

_____, thank you for
_____

_____, thank you for
_____

_____, thank you for
_____

_____, thank you for
_____

_____, thank you for
_____

_____, thank you for
_____

DAILY PRACTICE

Fill in the blanks with people, things, and events you are grateful for today. On some days you might feel like adding more—do so. On the days when it is more difficult to fill in the blanks, remember that you can be grateful for everybody and anything.

DATE: _____

I am grateful for _____

I am grateful for _____

I am grateful for _____

I am grateful for _____

I am grateful for _____

FIVE GRATITUDE INTENTIONS
Fill in the blanks with things you'd like to create in your daily life.

I am grateful for _____

I am grateful for _____

I am grateful for _____

I am grateful for _____

I am grateful for _____

Today I feel gratitude in my _____

CREATING MY DAILY GRATITUDE PRACTICE

Check off the type of gratitude statements you most enjoyed and see yourself doing regularly as part of your gratitude practice. These are reminders of the many different ways to express your gratitude. Also, commit to a time during the day you will set aside to write your gratitude list.

TYPES OF GRATITUDES	✓
Gratitudes from Today's Experiences	
Gratitude Intentions	
Kindness Gratitudes	
Forgiveness Gratitudes	
Being of Service Gratitudes	
Gratitude Meditations	
Gratitudes for the Hard Days	
Gratitudes for the Future	

TIME OF DAY _____

DAILY PRACTICE

Fill in the blanks with people, things, and events you are grateful for today. On some days you might feel like adding more—do so. On the days when it is more difficult to fill in the blanks, remember that you can be grateful for everybody and anything.

DATE:

I am grateful for _____

I am grateful for _____

I am grateful for _____

I am grateful for _____

I am grateful for _____

FIVE GRATITUDE INTENTIONS
Fill in the blanks with things you'd like to create in your daily life.

I am grateful for _____

I am grateful for _____

I am grateful for _____

I am grateful for _____

I am grateful for _____

Today I feel gratitude in my _____

GRATITUDE LETTER TO MYSELF

Write a letter to yourself about gratitude and what it means to you. Include those very special experiences you are grateful for, as well as the gratitude intentions you identified. Look into your heart and create the year that you desire as you look forward.

Dear Me,

_____

_____

_____

_____

_____

_____

_____

_____

_____

_____

_____

_____

_____

_____

_____

_____

_____

_____

I believe that gratitude is the best approach to life. When life is going well, it allows us to celebrate and magnify the goodness. When life is going badly, it provides a perspective by which we can view life in its entirety and not be overwhelmed by temporary experience. And this is what grateful people do. They have learned to transform adversity into opportunity no matter what happens, to see existence itself as a gift.

—Robert A. Emmons, PhD

RECOMMENDED READING

Arrien, Angeles. *Living in Gratitude: A Journey That Will Change Your Life*. Boulder, CO: Sounds True, 2011.

Davidson, Richard J., and Sharon Begley. *The Emotional Life of Your Brain: How Its Unique Patterns Affect the Way You Think, Feel, and Live—and How You Can Change Them*. New York: Hudson Street, 2012.

Emmons, Robert A. *The Little Book of Gratitude: Create a life of happiness and wellbeing by giving thanks*. London: Octopus Publishing, 2016.

Emmons, Robert A. *Thanks! How the New Science of Gratitude Can Make You Happier*. Boston: Houghton Mifflin, 2007.

Emmons, Robert. A., and Michael E. McCullough. *The Psychology of Gratitude*. New York: Oxford University Press, 2004.

Fogg, B.J. *Tiny Habits: The Small Changes That Change Everything*. Boston: Houghton Mifflin, 2019.

Hanson, Rick, and Forrest Hanson. *Resilient: How to Grow an Unshakable Core of Calm, Strength, and Happiness*. New York: Penguin, 2018.

Merzenich, Michael. *Soft-Wired: How the New Science of Brain Plasticity Can Change Your Life*. San Francisco: Parnassus, 2013.

ACKNOWLEDGMENTS

My deepest gratitude to everyone recognized here, who without their support I would never have undertaken the Resiliency Guide Series. First, I am grateful for my family. Christian, your resilience, kindness, and daily practices inspire me. I am grateful for your "one writer to another" encouragement, and your completely honest editorial comments. Having your support during this unforeseen and highly challenging year made it possible for me to fulfill my dream of sharing this life-altering information with as many people as possible. I am so grateful for you!

I am grateful for all my teachers during this 24-year healing journey. I am truly at a loss for words to describe the depth of my appreciation for you being there to instruct, assist, and remind me to practice. I am grateful for my yoga teacher. I am grateful for you never giving up on my healing goals when everyone else did. I am forever grateful for the dignity and respect with which you treat me. I am grateful for Pam Lanza & Glenn Hirsch who helped me become an artist when I could barely move my hands and arms. I miss you both, may you rest in peace. I am grateful for Dr. Maud Nerman and Adrienne Larkin for role modeling that healing is a lifelong journey and to never give up.

I am grateful for my friends and colleagues who stood with me during these many challenging years, enthusiastically encouraging my writing, art, and studies. I am grateful for my dear friend Faith Winthrop who told me this was going to happen. I will celebrate with you in my heart. I am grateful for my dear friends Laurie McFarlane, Aiko Morioka, and Cathy River for your unshakable support. I am grateful for Gordon Sumner, Karen Leveque, Matt Schwartz, and John Kirkpatrick, for supporting me in so many different ways. I am grateful for the people around the world who trust me daily with their joys, fears, accomplishments, hurts, and their hearts. I am honored to be of service to you!

I am grateful for those of you whose stellar work helped bring the Resiliency Guides into existence. I am grateful for Luke Schwartz, research assistant extraordinaire for expanding and coordinating my 20+ years of research sources. I am grateful for the amazing team at West Margin Press. I am grateful for Jen Newens for understanding my vision and providing the platform for this information to reach so many others. I am grateful for Olivia Ngai's detailed, precise, and inspired editing. I am grateful for Rachel Metzger's innovative designs capturing and reflecting the heart of these books. I am grateful for Angie Zbornik's strategic marketing ideas, innovative execution, support, and patience as I focused on the content. I deeply appreciate all your work. I am grateful for all of you!

ABOUT THE AUTHOR

Janine Wilburn is an award-winning artist, innovator, and writer. She has a master's degree in East West Psychology and is pursuing her PhD. For decades, Janine worked as a marketing professional, receiving recognition for her work with a Cannes Film Festival Bronze Lion, a Clio, and other awards, until a car accident changed her life. Suffering spinal damage, she needed to heal. Through her studies in neuroscience, neuroplasticity, yoga, and meditation, Janine persevered and developed resilience-building practices. The Resiliency Guides are the result of her research, experience, hope, and commitment to help others. Janine lives in San Francisco, California.

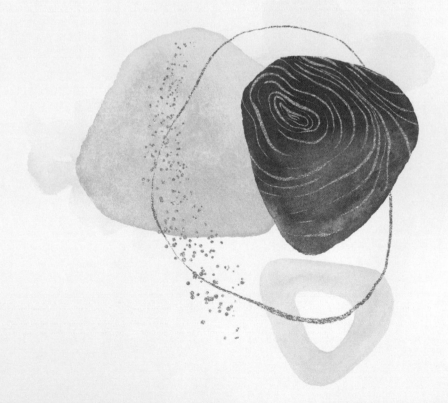

To everyone practicing gratitude or contemplating practicing gratitude during this most challenging time.

This book is not intended to diagnose or replace any medical advice or information. The publisher and author do not make any warranties about the completeness, reliability, or accuracy of the information in these pages. The publisher and author are not responsible and are not liable for any damages or negative consequences from any treatment, action, or application to any person reading or following the information in this book.

ISBN: 9781513289564

Printed in China
1 2 3 4 5

Published by West Margin Press

WEST MARGIN PRESS
WestMarginPress.com

Proudly distributed by Ingram Publisher Services

WEST MARGIN PRESS
Publishing Director: Jennifer Newens
Marketing Manager: Angela Zbornik
Project Specialist: Micaela Clark
Editor: Olivia Ngai
Design & Production: Rachel Lopez Metzger